25 Landmark Trials in Cardiology

25 LANDMARK TRIALS IN CARDIOLOGY

**Drs. Gabor Gyenes and Craig Butler
with Dr. Robert Welsh, Senior Editor**

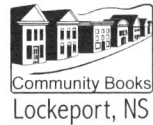

Community Books
Lockeport, NS

Copyright © 2006 Drs. Gabor Gyenes and Craig Butler
All rights reserved. Except for the quotation of short passages for review purposes, no part of this publication may be reproduced in any form without prior permission of the authors.

Design: Brenda Conroy
Printed and bound in Canada by
Hignell Printing, Winnipeg, MB
Published by Community Books
RR1, Lockeport, Nova Scotia, B0T 1L0
phone/fax: (902) 656-2223
email: kathleen.tudor@ns.sympatico.ca
www.selfpublishingspecialists.com

Copies of this book may be obtained from:
Gabor Gyenes MD PhD, Assistant Professor of Cardiology
University of Alberta Hospital, 2C2 Walter Mackenzie
Health Sciences Centre, Edmonton, AB
Canada T6G 2B7
Tel: (780) 407-7929, Fax: (780) 407-6918
ggyenes@cha.ab.ca
After November 2006, a mobile version of this book is available from www.skyscape.com

Library and Archives Canada Cataloguing in Publication

Gyenes, Gabor
   25 landmark trials in cardiology / Gabor Gyenes and Craig Butler.

Includes bibliographical references.
ISBN 1-896496-59-8

1. Heart—Diseases—Treatment—Evaluation—Handbooks, manuals, etc. 2. Clinical trials—Handbooks, manuals, etc. I. Butler, Craig R. (Craig Ronald), 1973- II. Title. III. Title: Twenty-five landmark trials in cardiology.

RC683.8.G94 2006   616.1'2060724   C2006-903536-9

Contents

Preface /7
Acronyms and Abbreviations /8

ST-elevation Myocardial Infarction (STEMI) Studies
    GISSI-1 /11
    GUSTO-1 /13
    CLARITY – TIMI 28 /15
    COMMIT – CCS 2 /17

Non-ST-elevation Myocardial Infarction (NSTEMI) Studies
    SYNERGY /19
    TACTICS-TIMI 18 /21
    CURE/ PCI-CURE /23

Atherosclerosis/Cardiovascular Protection
    FRAMINGHAM STUDY /25
    HOPE/MICRO-HOPE /27
    PEACE /29

Lipid Studies
    4S /31
    HPS /33
    PROVE-IT-TIMI 22 /35

Hypertension
    ALLHAT /38

Heart Failure/LV Dysfunction
    SOLVD /40
    DIG /42
    CHARM /43
    RALES /46
    MERIT-HF /48

Heart Failure/LV Dysfunction/Arrhythmias
    MADIT-II /50

Arrhythmias Including Atrial Fibrillation
    CAST /52
    AFASAK /53
    AFFIRM /55

Hormone Replacement Therapy
    WOMEN'S HEALTH INITIATIVE (WHI) /57

Diabetes and the Heart
    UKPDS-38 /59
    FURTHER UKPDS STUDIES /60

Additional References /61

Warning/Disclaimer

The purpose of this book is to highlight important trials in cardiovascular medicine, and it is not intended as a patient care reference. It is essential that physicians intending to apply trial results to actual patients first consult the original trial results referenced in this book. The authors assume no responsibility for the utilization of drugs or procedures recommended by the trials discussed in this book.

Acknowledgements

We are grateful to our families for putting up with our long working hours and for supporting us in doing what we love to do most.

We want to thank Dr. Lisa McKnight for the idea of the book and Dr. Benjamin Barankin for his insightful advice.

We also want to thank Brenda Conroy for the design of the book and both Brenda and Kathleen Tudor for being patient and helpful publishers beyond all expectations.

Senior Editor
Robert C. Welsh, MD, FRCPC, FACC

Dr. Robert Welsh received his Medical Doctorate from the University of Saskatchewan in 1993. Currently, he is Associate Professor and an academic Interventional Cardiologist at the University of Alberta Hospital in Edmonton. He is the Co-director of the University of Alberta Chest Pain Program, and he is the Director of the University of Alberta Cardiology Residency Training Program. He is also chair of Vital Heart Response; a regional reperfusion program for early treatment of STEMI patients.

He has been involved in several national and international multicenter trials. He has approximately 70 peer reviewed publications, journal reviews and abstracts.

Preface

A 56-year-old man presented the prior evening with a troponin positive acute coronary syndrome. After an uneventful night the patient's treatment strategy was being discussed at morning CCU rounds with due attention paid to 'evidenced based medicine.' The residents presented a variety of management strategies with enthusiastic defence of each proposal. "These are all reasonable plans," I interjected, "but what would the evidence have us do?" The response was considerably less enthusiastic. "Well there are only a thousand studies in cardiology, why is it so difficult to remember them all," I commented, trying to sound funny. "Yes there are a thousand studies so why isn't there a book on the most important ones?" asked one thoughtful resident.

This book was thus created in response to voiced frustrations among junior medicine, cardiology and off-service residents rotating through cardiology as well as non-cardiologist physicians who are overwhelmed by the sheer number of cardiology trials. After repeated requests for references of 'just the important trials' or 'just the trials that changed practice,' Craig and I decided to compile a user-friendly quick-reference guide of the '25 trials' that had the biggest impact on clinical practice across the breadth of cardiovascular medicine.

Naturally, the most difficult and contentious part of writing this handbook was to select a limited number of landmark studies that really changed the way cardiology is practised today. We thought long and hard about our selections and sought thoughtful opinions from our colleagues such as Dr. Rob Welsh, who himself has been involved in numerous international studies, and ultimately decided upon the list published here. We really tried to key in on trials that residents and non-cardiologists need to know about. We hope the addition of our editorial remarks will facilitate understanding by placing each trial in context and emphasizing important strengths or limitations in the interpretation of trial results. We used published editorial remarks, consensus opinions as well as our personal judgment to give a balanced view — you will be the judge of how we succeeded.

If you want to order copies of this book or have any comments or suggestions for the future updates, please contact Dr. Gabor Gyenes at ggyenes@cha.ab.ca. The digital version will be available after November 2006 from www.skyscape.com. We hope this book will be a useful and relevant companion to you.

Gabor Gyenes

Acronyms and Abbreviations

ACS – acute coronary syndrome
AE – adverse events
(A)MI – (acute) myocardial infarction
ARR – absolute risk reduction
CCB – calcium channel blocker
CHD – coronary heart disease
CVD – cardiovascular disease
CI – confidence interval
CK – creatine kinase
CRF – chronic renal failure
c/w – compared with
DM – diabetes mellitus
EF – ejection fraction
GP IIb/IIIa – glycoprotein IIb/IIIa antagonist
HF – heart failure
HTN – hypertension
ICD (or AICD) – (automatic) implantable cardioverter-defibrillator
IHD – ischemic heart disease
IVUS – intravascular ultrasonography
JACC – Journal of the American College of Cardiology
LV – left ventricle or left ventricular
LBBB – left bundle branch block
LE – liver enzymes
LVD – left ventricular dysfunction
LVEF – left ventricular ejection fraction
Non-STEMI - myocardial infarction without ST-elevation
NS – not significant
NSR – normal sinus rhythm
NSTE ACS – non-ST elevation acute coronary syndrome
NYHA – New York Heart Association (HF classification)
od – once daily
OR – odds ratio
PCI – percutaneous coronary intervention
PVD – peripheral vascular disease
RCT – randomized controlled trial
RR(R) – relative risk (reduction)
SK - Streptokinase
STEMI – ST-elevation myocardial infarction
TC – total cholesterol
t-PA – tissue plasminogen activator
UA – unstable angina
ULN – upper limit of normal

The Studies

ST-elevation Myocardial Infarction (STEMI) Studies
GISSI-1

Gruppo Italiano per lo Studio della Streptochinasi Nell'Infarto Miocardico
Lancet 1986;327:397-402 and
Lancet 1987;330:871-874.

Study Question
Does Streptokinase (SK) reduce morbidity and mortality in myocardial infarction?

Methods
Multicenter non-blinded randomized trial of 11,806 patients with an acute myocardial infarction (both ST-elevation and ST-depression) within 12 hours of symptoms.
Patients were randomized to 1.5 million units of streptokinase (SK) vs. placebo. In addition all patients received "usual practice" of each recruiting hospital.

Results
Concomitant Therapy: Heparin iv = 21%, ASA = 13%, Beta blocker = 8%. There were no significant differences between SK and placebo groups with respect to concomitant treatments.

21 day mortality
SK vs. Placebo:
All Patients:	10.7% vs. 13%	RR 0.81	p=0.0002
ST depression:	20.5% vs. 16.3%		p=NS
Killip Class IV:	69.9% vs. 70.1%		p=NS

21 day mortality benefit stratified by time between onset of pain and SK infusion
<1 hr RR 0.49	(95% CI 0.34-0.69, p=0.0001)
≤3 hr RR 0.74	(95% CI 0.63-0.87, p=0.0005)
3-6 hr RR 0.80	(95% CI 0.66-0.98, p=0.03)
6-9 hr RR 0.87	(95% CI 0.64-1.19, p=NS)
9-12 hr RR 1.19	(95% CI 0.75-1.87, p=NS)

12 month total mortality
SK vs. Placebo:
17.2% vs. 19.0%   RR 0.90 (95% CI 0.84-0.97, p=0.008)

ST-elevation Myocardial Infarction (STEMI) Studies

12 month total mortality benefit stratified by time between onset of pain and SK infusion

    0-3 h: 15.1% vs. 17.3%   RR 0.89 (95% CI 0.79-1.0, p=0.02)
    3-6 h: 18.3% vs. 21.2%   RR 0.87 (95% CI 0.76-0.99, p=0.02)
    0-1 h: 12.9% vs. 21.2%   RR 0.61 (95% CI 0.47-0.78, p=0.00001)

Adverse Events
    Major bleeding attributable to SK: 0.3% at 21 days; stroke: 0.2%.

Conclusion

1.5 million units of SK is a safe and effective treatment for AMI if it can be given within 6 hours of symptom onset.

Perspective

GISSI-1 was the first large scale study to demonstrate the benefit of fibrinolysis with SK over placebo, demonstrating enhanced short-term and long-term mortality. This trial also underlined the importance of administering reperfusion therapy quickly after symptom onset as evidenced by the fact that the largest mortality reduction was seen in those treated earliest. This trial solidified reperfusion therapy for the treatment of acute ST elevation myocardial infarction and provided the groundwork for further investigations into reperfusion strategies.

    The ISIS-2 trial[1] provided the next important step showing the additive benefit of aspirin to SK. This study demonstrated that aspirin alone or SK alone provided similar benefit compared to placebo, but the combination enhanced outcomes in an additive fashion.

1. ISIS-2: *Lancet* 1986;328:57-66.

GUSTO-1

An International Randomized Trial Comparing Four Thrombolytic Strategies for Acute Myocardial Infarction: The Global Utilization of Streptokinase and Tissue Plasminogen Activator (t-PA) for Occluded Coronary Arteries Investigators.
New England Journal of Medicine 1993;329:673-682.

Study Question
Multicenter, open label trial to assess 30 day mortality and safety profile of four different thrombolytic protocols in the management of acute STEMI.

Methods
41,021 patients with STEMI defined as: 20 minutes of chest pain presenting within 6 hours of onset and ST elevation (1 mm in two limb leads, 2 mm in two precordial leads)
Patients were randomized to one of four groups:
1) Streptokinase (SK) + heparin sc, 2) SK + heparin iv, 3) t-PA + heparin iv, 4) t-PA + SK + heparin iv.

Results

t-PA vs. Both SK Groups:
24 hour mortality:	2.3% vs. 2.9%	(p=0.005)
30 day mortality:	6.3% vs. 7.3%	(p=0.001)
Hemorrhagic stroke:	0.72% vs. 0.52%	(p=0.03)
Allergic reactions:	1.6% vs. 5.8%	(p<0.001)

t-PA vs. SK + t-PA:
30 day mortality:	6.3% vs. 7.0%	(p=0.04)
Hemorrhagic stroke:	0.72% vs. 0.94%	(p=0.03)

t-PA + SK vs. Both SK Groups:
30 day mortality:	7.0% vs. 7.3%	(p=0.352)
Hemorrhagic stroke:	0.94% vs. 0.52%	(p=0.001)

Absolute mortality benefit for t-PA vs. SK was 1.0% (p=0.001).

Pre-specified subgroup analyses showed t-PA was not better than SK in:
  Patients >75 years
  Patients with inferior infarctions
  Patients presenting >4 hours after symptom onset

ST-elevation Myocardial Infarction (STEMI) Studies

Conclusion

t-PA has a small but important mortality benefit compared to SK in the treatment of acute STEMI.

Perspective

This trial demonstrated the mortality advantage of the more fibrin-specific t-PA versus SK. This established t-PA as the gold standard reperfusion therapy with a 1% mortality reduction compared to SK albeit at an increased risk of bleeding. Over the next decade intense investigation interrogating alterations of the native t-PA molecule in attempts to create better fibrinolytic agents followed. This has led to the development of single bolus tenecteplase (TNK), which has been shown equivalent to t-PA, and double bolus reteplase (r-PA), as well as other agents that failed to pass the rigours of scientific investigations.

CLARITY – TIMI 28

Clopidogrel as Adjunctive Reperfusion Therapy – Thrombolysis in Myocardial Infarction 28.
New England Journal of Medicine 2005;352:1179-1189.

Study Question
Does the addition of clopidogrel to thrombolytic therapy improve patency in the infarct-related artery in STEMI?

Methods
Multicenter international randomized placebo controlled trial that enrolled 3,491 patients, 18-75 years of age with an ST-elevation MI.
Patients were randomized to clopidogrel (300 mg loading dose, followed by 75 mg once daily) or placebo.
All patients also received: fibrinolysis, aspirin, and heparin. All patients had coronary angiography within 48-192 hours of admission.

Results
Primary endpoint: Composite of an occluded infarct-related artery on angiography or death or recurrent myocardial infarction before angiography.

Clopidogrel vs. Placebo:
Primary endpoint: 15% vs. 21.7% RR 0.64 (95% CI 0.53-0.76, p<0.001)
ARR: 6.7%

At 30 days:
CV death/MI/Urgent Revascularization: 11.6% vs. 14.1% RR 0.80
(95% CI 0.65-0.97, p=0.03).

Major bleeding and intracranial hemorrhage was not different between groups.

Conclusion
In patients ≤75 years of age with ST-elevation MI, the addition of clopidogrel to the standard fibrinolytic regimen improves the patency rate of the infarct-related artery and reduces ischemic complications significantly.

Perspective
CLARITY TIMI 28 investigated the impact of additional antiplatelet therapy in combination with standard antithrombotics and fibrinolytics. This followed on the heels of a host of investigations into administration of potent GPIIb/IIIa receptor blockers in conjunction with various fibrinolytic agents and doses, which demonstrated increased risk with no benefit. In contrast, the addition of clopidogrel to aspirin, antithrombotic and standard fibrinolytic therapy

ST-elevation Myocardial Infarction (STEMI) Studies

demonstrated enhanced patency of the infarct artery with fewer complications prior to an angiogram completed at two to three days post-MI. Although the more standard composite clinical endpoint of death, recurrent MI or urgent revascularization, favoured clopidogrel therapy, the trial was not powered to detect a mortality benefit.

These benefits were achieved without an increased risk of bleeding in this relatively low risk and young population with effectively managed anticoagulation strategy.

The much larger COMMIT-CCS 2 trial[2] conducted in China, tested the addition of clopidogrel without a loading dose (75 mg once daily) in 45,852 predominantly STEMI patients. This trial demonstrated a significant though modest mortality reduction consistent with the results of CLARITY TIMI 28.

2. COMMIT-CCS 2 – clopidogrel randomization: *Lancet* 2005;366:1607-21.

COMMIT – CCS 2

Clopidogrel and Metoprolol in Myocardial Infarction Trial
Lancet 2005;366:1622-32.

Study Question
Do metoprolol and clopidogrel independently reduce adverse outcomes in acute coronary syndromes?

Methods
Double blinded randomized trial with a 2x2 factorial design of 45,852 patients within 24 hours of presentation with a suspected acute MI (93% STEMI or bundle branch block, 7% non-STEMI). Patients were randomized to receive clopidogrel vs. placebo and metoprolol vs. placebo. (The clopidogrel arm is discussed on page 15 with the CLARITY Study.)
Patients were randomization to Metoprolol up to 15 mg iv, then 200 mg po daily or placebo until discharge or up to 4 weeks in hospital.

Results
Primary endpoints: (1) composite of death, reinfarction, or cardiac arrest; (2) death from any cause.

Metoprolol vs. Placebo:
Death/MI/Cardiac arrest: 9.4% vs. 9.9%   (p=0.1)
All cause mortality: OR 0.99 (95% CI 0.92-1.05, p=0.69)
Reinfarction: OR 0.82 (95% CI 0.72-0.92, p=0.001)
VF: OR 0.83 (95% CI 0.75-0.93, p=0.001)
Cardiogenic shock*:   OR 1.30 (95% CI 1.19-1.41, p<0.00001)

*1.1% increased absolute risk for cardiogenic shock was mainly seen within 24 hours of admission.
Metoprolol therapy showed significant harm during days 0-1 and significant benefits thereafter.

Conclusion
"The use of early β-blocker therapy in acute MI reduces the risks of reinfarction and ventricular fibrillation, but increases the risk of cardiogenic shock, especially during the first day or so after admission." Consequently, beta blocker therapy at the doses applied in this trial should be given cautiously particularly in the first 24 hours after an AMI.

Perspective
This beta blocker mega trial has identified the importance of ongoing scientific investigation and the importance of revisiting recommendations that are based on dated data and/or statistical trends. The aggressive dosing strategy

used within this trial is not fully consistent with the current Guidelines' recommendations and it is inconsistent with most physicians' clinical practice. The ongoing judicious use of intravenous and oral beta blockers in appropriate clinical situations remains grounded on scientific evidence and will likely remain incorporated into subsequent clinical guidelines.

Non-ST-elevation Myocardial Infarction (NSTEMI) Studies

SYNERGY

Enoxaparin vs. Unfractionated Heparin in High-risk Patients with Non-ST-Segment Elevation Acute Coronary Syndromes Managed with an Intended Early Invasive Strategy. The Superior Yield of the New Strategy of Enoxaparin, Revascularization and Glycoprotein IIb/IIIa Inhibitors Study.
JAMA 2004;292:45-54.

Study Question
Which heparin has the greatest effect on lowering adverse outcomes in acute coronary syndromes managed with an early invasive approach?

Methods
Randomized trial of 10,027 adults with high risk NSTEMI (age >60 yrs, positive cardiac markers or ST segment changes).
Patients were randomized to either enoxaparin 1 mg/kg/12 hrs or unfractionated heparin (bolus of 60 U/kg [max. 5000 U] and 12 U/kg/hr [max. 1000 U/h]).
The study protocol dictated mandatory cardiac catheterization (with possible PCI) within 24 hours of admission.

Results
Enoxaparin vs. Unfractionated Heparin:

All cause mortality or MI:	14% vs. 14.5%	(p=NS)
Abrupt vessel occlusion:	1.3% vs. 1.7%	(p=NS)
Failed PCI:	3.6% vs. 3.4%	(p=NS)
Emergency CABG:	0.3% vs. 0.3%	(p=NS)

Subgroup analysis:
75% of patients had been started on a heparin prior to enrollment. Patients without pre-randomization antithrombin therapy and patients who were randomized to the same antithrombin therapy they received pre-enrollment had fewer primary endpoints (death or MI at 30 days) when randomized to enoxaparin therapy (13.5% vs. 14.2% RR=0.82, 95% CI 0.72-0.94) compared to "pretreated and crossover" patients (i.e., started on enoxaparin then randomized to unfractionated heparin iv).

Non-ST-elevation Myocardial Infarction (NSTEMI) Studies

Primary safety outcome: major bleeding or stroke
Enoxaparin vs. Unfractionated Heparin:
TIMI major bleeding: 9.1% vs. 7.6%   (p=0.008)
TIMI minor bleeding: 12.5% vs. 12.3% (p=0.8)
No increase in intracranial hemorrhage, transfusions, or hemodynamic compromise.

Conclusion
Enoxaparin has similar efficacy to unfractionated heparin, however its convenience is at the expense of a small increase in major bleeding complications.

Perspective
This trial was designed to confirm the perceived advantage of enoxaparin over unfractionated heparin in a large population of high risk NSTE ACS patients. Despite the prior promising results (e.g., FRISC II[3], ESSENCE[4], TIMI 11B[5], etc.) this mega trial demonstrated no advantage of the low molecular weight heparin enoxaparin in high risk patients with early cardiac catheterization and PCI within 24 hours from admission. Multiple secondary analyses of this trial have been undertaken, demonstrating a host of interesting, albeit hypothesis-generating, points for discussion. Firstly, within this trial a substantial portion of patients were pre-treated with anticoagulation before being randomized. When only those patients who were "anticoagulation-naïve" or on consistent anticoagulation therapy were assessed, the predicted advantage of enoxaparin over unfractionated heparin was demonstrated. Secondly, in countries like Canada, where time to cardiac catheterization was more prolonged, the benefit of enoxaparin was again suggested. Thirdly, there was a strong suggestion that crossing over from one anticoagulant to the other was associated with increased bleeding and ischemic complications.

Although this trial failed to prove the advantage of enoxaparin, it did clarify the importance of consistent anticoagulation with a single agent from the time of admission to hospital through cardiac catheterization, percutaneous coronary intervention, medical stabilization and discharge.

3. FRISC II: *Lancet* 1999;354:708-15.
4. ESSENCE: *NEJM* 1997;337:447-52.
5. TIMI 11B: *Circulation* 1999;100:1593-1601.

TACTICS-TIMI 18

Comparison of Early Invasive and Conservative Strategies in Patients with Unstable Coronary Syndromes Treated with Glycoprotein IIb/IIIa Inhibitor Tirofiban.
Treat Angina with Aggrastat and Determine Cost of Therapy with an Invasive or Conservative Strategy – Thrombolysis in Myocardial Infarction 18 Study.
New England Journal of Medicine 2001;344:1879-1887.

Study Question
Does early invasive therapy reduce adverse outcomes compared to conservative therapy in a population of acute coronary syndrome patients treated with tirofiban?

Methods
Randomized controlled trial of 2,220 adults with Acute Coronary Syndromes who were randomized to early invasive (coronary catheterization <48 hours) or conservative management (coronary catheterization only if recurrent angina or positive non-invasive testing).
All patients received ASA, heparin, and tirofiban.

Results
Early Invasive vs. Conservative:

6 month death/MI/re-hospitalization:	15.9% vs. 19.4%	(p=0.025)
6 month death or MI:	7.3% vs. 9.5%	(p<0.05)

Benefit was seen at 1 week, 30 days and 6 months.

Subgroups:
Early Invasive vs. Conservative (Death/MI/re-hospitalization):

Positive troponin:	16.4% vs. 24.5%	(p<0.05)
ST segment change:	16.4% vs. 26.3%	(p<0.05)
High risk by TIMI score:	19.5% vs. 30.6%	(p<0.05)

Conclusion
NSTEMI patients who received coronary catheterization and possible revascularization within 48 hours along with tirofiban treatment had lower rates of death or MI or repeat hospitalization. Subgroup analysis suggests that higher risk patients (elevated cardiac enzymes, ST segment change on EKG, and TIMI risk scores ≥ 3) receive the most benefit.

Perspective
There is a long running debate about which NSTEMI patients should have early angiography versus medical management with subsequent angiography if indicated on the basis of clinical deterioration or results of non-invasive

Non-ST-elevation Myocardial Infarction (NSTEMI) Studies

testing. TACTICS TIMI 18 is considered by many to be strong evidence for early catheterization in NSTE ACS, in particular for patients with high risk features.

The study was impressive because 51% of the patients on the conservative arm had an angiogram (51% cross-over), 36% had revascularization and despite this the invasive arm (97% angiography and 61% revascularization) still demonstrated significant benefits.

The recently published ICTUS[6] trial showed no benefit of an early invasive approach in contrast to TACTICS TIMI 18. ISAR-COOL[7], which used aggressive antithrombotic management in both arms with early angiography versus later angiography, was supportive of the results of TACTICS TIMI18. The logical equipoise between past and current data suggests that in true high risk NSTE ACS patients rapid access to cardiac catheterization and appropriate revascularization appears beneficial, as long as this can be achieved between 24-48 hours. Many real life patients do not qualify for early cardiac catheterization and remain stable in hospital such that a more conservative approach with non-invasive testing guiding therapy with cardiac catheterization would also be acceptable.

6. ICTUS: *NEJM* 2005;353:1095-1104.
7. ISAR-COOL: *JAMA* 2003;290:1593-9.

CURE

Clopidogrel in Unstable Angina to Prevent Recurrent Events.
New England Journal of Medicine 2001;345:494-502.

PCI-CURE

Effects of Pretreatment with Clopidogrel and Aspirin Followed by Long-term Therapy in Patients Undergoing Percutaneous Coronary Intervention.
Lancet 2001;358:527-533.

Study Question
CURE: Does the addition of clopidogrel reduce adverse events in NSTEMI?
PCI CURE: Does clopidogrel treatment prior to PCI and up to 12 months after PCI prevent more adverse outcomes than 4 weeks of clopidogrel post PCI?

Methods
A randomized, placebo controlled multicenter trial involving 12,562 patients with non-ST-elevation MI who had presented within 24 hours after the onset of symptoms. Patients were randomized to clopidogrel (300 mg as a loading dose followed by 75 mg once daily) or placebo for 3 to 12 months. All patients received aspirin.
The study was conducted in centers where the early invasive approach was not routinely used and GP IIb/IIIa use was discouraged.
PCI-CURE: a sub-study of 2,658 patients with non-ST-elevation ACS undergoing PCI. After PCI, >80% patients in both groups received open-label clopidogrel for about 4 weeks.

Results
Clopidogrel vs. Placebo:
CV death/MI/Stroke:	9.3% vs. 11.4%	($p<0.001$)
CV death/MI/Stroke/refractory angina:	16.5% vs. 18.8%	($p<0.001$)

Safety outcome
Clopidogrel vs. Placebo:
Major bleeding:	3.7% vs. 2.7%	($p=0.001$)
Life-threatening bleeding:	2.1% vs. 1.8%	($p=0.13$)
Hemorrhagic stroke:	0.1% vs. 0.1%	($p=NS$)
Major bleeding post bypass:	1.3% vs. 1.1%	($p=NS$)

PCI-CURE
Clopidogrel vs. Placebo:

30 day CV death/MI/urgent revascularization:	4.5% vs. 6.4%	(p=0.03)
CV death or MI:	2.9% vs. 4.4%	(p=0.04)
CV death:	1.1% vs. 1.0%	(p=NS)
8 month CV death/MI/revascularization:	18.3% vs. 21.7%	(p=0.03)

Overall (before and after PCI) CV death or MI: RRR 0.69 (95% CI 0.54-0.87, p=0.002).

Adverse Events
No difference in major bleeding between groups (p=0.64)

Conclusion
The antiplatelet agent clopidogrel reduced adverse events in patients with NSTE ACS. The risk of major bleeding in the main study was increased among patients treated with clopidogrel.

Perspective
The CURE trial demonstrated that the combined antiplatelet therapy of aspirin and clopidogrel, in addition to heparin, significantly reduced the composite endpoint. The benefit of this dual therapy occurred early and appeared sustained out to the end of the trial. This trial changed our baseline antithrombotic therapy in documented ACS patients to include aspirin, clopidogrel and therapeutic anticoagulation (unfractionated heparin or enoxaparin). The optimal combination of therapies, especially the role of GP IIb/IIIa drugs outside of the cath lab continues to be debated. However, the recently published ISAR-REACT 2[8] trial in high risk patients continues to show benefit of glycoprotein IIb/IIIa receptor blockers on top of the above-mentioned new baseline therapy.

PCI-CURE was an observational sub-study based on non-randomized interventions driven by refractory symptoms or recurrent adverse cardiac events. Within the study, GP IIb/IIIa use was discouraged and early invasive strategy was not mandated. Therefore, the CURE/PCI-CURE study results may not be widely applicable to current ACS management in North America.

Despite the above controversies clopidogrel therapy is gaining wide acceptance in the treatment of NSTE ACS. As well, the number of indications for clopidogrel therapy continues to grow both in the treatment of AMI (with or without PCI) and chronic atherosclerotic disease and ultimately it could even replace aspirin were it not for its high cost.

8. ISAR-REACT 2: *JAMA* 2006;295:1531:8.

Atherosclerosis/Cardiovascular Protection
FRAMINGHAM STUDY

Framingham risk score reference: *JAMA* 2001;285:2486.
Recent Framingham references: *Int J Cardiol* 2005;104:228;
Circulation 2005;112:1113-20; *Circulation* 2005;112:969-75,
and *Diabetologia* 2005;48:1492-5.
Framingham Offspring publications: *Am J Epidemiol* 2005;162:644-53;
Clin Cardiol 2005;28:247-51; *Am J Cardiol* 2004;94:1561-3,
Circulation 2004;110:380-5, and *JAMA 2005;294:3117-23*.

Study Question
Are there risk factors for atherosclerosis? What is the natural history of atherosclerotic vascular disease?

Methods
This is an ongoing epidemiological study of a small town called Framingham, Massachusetts, which started in 1948 and is sponsored by the National Heart Lung and Blood Institute. Originally, it enrolled 5,209 healthy residents between 30 and 60 years of age.
The Framingham Offspring study was initiated in 1971, and it recruited 5,124 children (and their spouses) of the original cohort.

Results
The study resulted in more than a 1,000 papers.
Some of its key findings regarding cardiovascular risk factors such as age, gender, blood pressure, and smoking were incorporated in the Framingham risk score, which is widely used to assess an individual's cardiovascular risks in the following 10 years. Family history of cardiovascular disease was not incorporated in this score; however, it was addressed by the Framingham Offspring study that showed:

Sibling CV disease (brothers <55, sisters <65 yr):
    Age- and sex-adjusted   OR 1.55   (95% CI 1.19-2.03)
    Risk factor-adjusted   OR 1.45   (95% CI 1.10-1.91).
Adjusted for sibling and parental CVD with both parents included in the study:
    OR for sibling   CVD 1.99   (95% CI 1.32-3.00)
    OR for parental   CVD 1.45   (95% CI 1.02-2.05).

Perspective

This study coined the term "risk factors" and helped establish the connection between atherosclerosis and high total and LDL-cholesterol levels, as well as low HDL-cholesterol levels, smoking, hypertension and diabetes mellitus.

Before the Framingham Study atherosclerosis was thought to be a part of normal aging and as such was considered non-modifiable. It was also the first major cardiovascular study to recruit female participants.

The Framingham Offspring study illustrated that a positive family history for coronary disease was not as significant as was previously thought.

The most frequently mentioned criticism of the study is that it almost exclusively investigated a Caucasian population. Therefore, recently, 500 members of Framingham's minority community have been recruited to participate in the Omni Study. Another large epidemiological study, the INTERHEART[9] included non-Caucasian populations and will most likely serve as a major reference paper in this regard.

9. INTERHEART: *Lancet* 2004;364:937-952.

HOPE/MICROHOPE

Effects of an ACE Inhibitor, Ramipril, on Cardiovascular Events in High-risk Patients.
The Heart Outcomes Prevention Study
New England Journal of Medicine 2000;342:145-153,
and *New England Journal of Medicine* 2000;342:154-160.

MICRO-HOPE

Lancet 2000; 355:253-259.

Study Question
Does the ACE inhibitor ramipril reduce cardiovascular events in high risk patients with normal ejection fractions?

Methods
Randomized double blind trial of 9,297 high risk patients over the age of 55 with an LV ejection fraction >40%. High risk was defined as one of the following: 1) History of CHD 2) History of stroke 3) History of PVD 4) DM + 1 other CV risk factor.
Patients were randomized according to a 2 x 2 factorial design comparing ramipril 10 mg vs. placebo as well as vitamin E vs. placebo. Patients were followed for 5-years.
MICRO-HOPE, a sub-study focusing on 3,577 diabetic patients treated with ramipril vs. placebo with respect to macro and renovascular outcomes. It was stopped early (4.5 years) due to highly significant and wide ranging benefit of ramipril treatment.

Results
Baseline BP (139/79 mmHg) not different between groups.
Ramipril lowered BP by 3/2 mmHg compared to placebo.

Primary endpoint: composite of CV death, MI or stroke.
Ramipril vs. Placebo:
Death/MI/stroke:	14% vs. 17.8%	($p<0.001$)
Overall mortality:	10.4% vs. 12.2%	($p<0.005$)
Myocardial infarction:	9.9% vs. 12.3%	($p<0.001$)
Stroke:	3.4% vs. 4.9%	($p<0.001$)
New diagnosis of diabetes:	3.6% vs. 5.4%	($p<0.001$)

Benefits were seen after 1 year of treatment.

MICRO-HOPE
Ramipril vs. Placebo:

Death/MI/stroke:	15.3% vs. 19.8%	(p=0.0004)
Cardiovascular mortality:	6.2% vs. 9.7%	(p=0.0001)
MI:	10.2% vs. 12.9%	(p=0.01)
CHF:	11% vs. 13.3%	(p=0.02)
Stroke:	4.2% vs. 6.1%	(p=0.007)
Overt nephropathy:	6.5% vs. 8.4%	(p=0.03)

Conclusion

"Ramipril significantly reduces the rates of death, MI, and stroke in a broad range of high-risk patients who are not known to have a low LV ejection fraction or heart failure." Vitamin E on the other hand did not affect cardiovascular outcomes in this patient population.

Perspective

This was the first trial to show the benefit of ACE inhibitors in patients with normal ejection fraction. HOPE demonstrated an impressive reduction in microvascular and macrovascular events with ramipril in all of the subgroups. After the release of HOPE, ramipril and ACE inhibitors in general quickly became routine therapy for vascular disease.

HOPE was also the first study to indicate that ramipril may prevent the development of new diabetes.

Some critics claim that it was the BP reduction in the ramipril group, not the drug itself that accounted for the observed benefits. However, previous hypertension trials required much larger reductions in blood pressure to achieve a similar magnitude of effect.

Despite the benefits of ramipril within the HOPE trial population, recent trials have brought into question the utilization of ACE inhibitors in certain populations with atherosclerotic disease. Specifically, the recently presented IMAGINE[10] trial demonstrating no benefit of randomization to ACE inhibitor following coronary artery bypass grafting brings into question the necessity of ACE inhibitors in absolutely all patient populations with coronary artery disease. See also comments on the PEACE study (page 29).

HOPE (as well as the Heart Protection Study – see page 33) just as convincingly showed that Vitamin E was not effective in preventing hard cardiovascular endpoints.

10. IMAGINE: presented at the European Society of Cardiology Congress, in Stockholm, Sweden, August 2005.

Atherosclerosis/Cardiovascular Protection

PEACE

Prevention of Events with Angiotensin Converting Enzyme Inhibition Trial
New England Journal of Medicine 2004;351:2058-68.

Study Question
Does the angiotensin converting enzyme inhibitor trandolapril reduce cardiovascular events in patients with coronary disease who are treated with current conventional therapy?

Methods
Randomized double blind placebo controlled trial of 8,290 adults over 50 years of age who had stable CHD and preserved EF (>40%). Patients were randomized to trandolapril 4 mg daily or placebo. Median follow up was 4.8 years.

Results
Randomization: more patients had diabetes in the trandolapril group
   (18% vs. 16% p<0.05).
Concomitant medication use between groups was not different
   (ASA 90%, statin 70%, beta blocker 60%).
Mean blood pressure reduction on trandolapril vs. placebo
   4.4 mmHg vs. 1.4 mmHg (p<0.001).
75% compliance with trandolapril therapy at 3 years.
8% crossover ACE inhibitor use in placebo group at 3 years.

Primary endpoint: CV death, MI, or revascularization.
   Trandolapril vs. Placebo:
   CV death/MI/Urgent revascularization: 21.9% vs. 22.5% (p=0.43)
   MI: 5.3% vs. 5.3 % (p=1.00)
   Stroke: 1.7% vs. 2.2%   (p=0.09)

Conclusion
Treatment with trandolapril 4mg daily does not further reduce cardiovascular endpoints in a population of patients with stable CHD, preserved LVEF, who had a low risk for recurrent cardiovascular events.

Perspective
It was surprising that PEACE failed to show prevention of macrovascular events with ACE inhibitor treatment considering that two other similarly designed trials of ACE inhibitors (HOPE and EUROPA[11]) showed significant benefits. When the baseline characteristics of HOPE, EUROPA and PEACE were compared it was apparent that the PEACE trial had a higher prevalence of revascularization procedures and a greater proportion of patients receiving lipid lowering therapy. The net effect was that the cardiovascular event rates of

the placebo group in the PEACE trial were almost as low as that of the general population, making it very difficult to show further significant benefits. PEACE ultimately was stopped early as it became clear that the very small effect size of trandolapril therapy would have required many more patients to show significance.

The meta-analysis[12] of PEACE, HOPE and EUROPA still showed significant benefit with ACE inhibitor therapy although this was predominantly driven by HOPE.

Nevertheless, results of PEACE and IMAGINE[10] – another neutral ACE inhibitor trial – have significantly tempered the enthusiasm for ACE inhibitors that the HOPE results had generated. The two neutral trials have illustrated that ACE inhibitor treatment on top of other treatment modalities such as complete revascularization and aggressive lipid-lowering currently may be of less benefit than prior studies had indicated. However, there remains a broad spectrum of patients in whom ACE-inhibition provides significant benefits such as patients with HF/LVD, AMI, DM, HTN, CRF and in some patients, vascular protection.

10. IMAGINE: presented at the European Society of Cardiology Congress, in Stockholm, Sweden, August, 2005
11. EUROPA: *Lancet* 2003;362:782-788.
12. Yusuf: *N Engl J Med*. 2005;352:937-8.

Lipid Studies

4S

Randomized Trial of Cholesterol Lowering in 4,444 Patients with Coronary Heart Disease: The Scandinavian Simvastatin Survival Study
Lancet 1994;344:1383-1389 and *Lancet* 1995;345:1274-1275.

Study Question
Does simvastatin reduce mortality in patients with coronary disease and hyperlipidemia?

Methods
Double blind randomized placebo controlled trial of 4,444 patients with elevated cholesterol (total cholesterol 5.5-8.0 mmol/L) and a history of coronary disease defined as angina or prior MI.
Patients were randomized to simvastatin (S) 20 mg (titrated to achieve a TC<5.2 mmol/L) vs. placebo (Pl).
Median follow up was 5.4 years.

Results
Simvastatin dose: 20 mg (63%), 40 mg (37%)
Simvastatin reduced LDL by 38% and increased HDL by 8%.

> *Simvastatin vs. Placebo:*
> All cause mortality: 8.2% vs. 11.5% RR 0.70 (95% CI 0.58-0.85, p=0.0003)
> Coronary mortality: 5% vs. 8.5% RR 0.58 (95% CI 0.46-0.73)
> Non-CV mortality: NS
> ≥1 major coronary event: 19% vs. 28% RR 0.66 (95% CI 0.59-0.75, p<0.00001)

Mortality benefit was evident after 1.5 years of treatment.
Reduction in coronary events was evident after 1 year.
Benefits were the same regardless of baseline cholesterol levels.

Adverse Events
Simvastatin vs. Placebo:
Rhabdomyolysis: 1 vs. 0 case
CK elevation >10x ULN: 6 vs. 1 cases

Conclusion

Long-term cholesterol lowering with simvastatin is safe and effective in achieving a significant reduction in both coronary morbidity and mortality.

Perspective

Prior to the 4S trial there was no conclusive evidence that reducing cholesterol would reduce cardiovascular mortality. The results of the 4S trial established LDL lowering as one of the cornerstones of cardiovascular disease prevention. By reducing LDL cholesterol by 38%, simvastatin lowered all cause mortality by an impressive 30%. There are very few therapies in cardiology that are this effective at lowering mortality. This trial provided the groundwork for a host of trials that followed that tested the impact of lipid reduction across a broad spectrum of patient populations with CVD.

HPS

MRC/BHF Heart Protection Study of Cholesterol Lowering with Simvastatin in 20,536 High-risk Individuals: A Randomized Placebo Controlled Trial
Lancet 2002;360:7-22, and *Lancet* 2003;361:2005-16 (Diabetic sub-study).

Study Question
Does simvastatin, vitamins or both prevent cardiovascular outcomes in individuals with relatively normal cholesterol levels, but with documented vascular disease or multiple CV risk factors?

Methods
Double blind randomized placebo controlled trial with a 2 x 2 factorial design of 20,536 adults with stable CAD, PVD, or Type II DM.
Patients were randomized according to a 2 x 2 factorial design to:
    simvastatin 40 mg or placebo, and
    vitamins (vit E 600 mg, vit C 250 mg, β-carotene 20 mg) or placebo.
Five years of follow up.

Results
Incidence of major outcomes
Simvastatin vs. Placebo:

All-cause mortality:	12.9% vs. 14.7% (p=0.0003)
Cardiac mortality:	5.7% vs. 6.9% (p=0.0005)
Nonfatal MI or CV death:	8.7% vs. 11.8% (p=0.0001)
Stroke:	4.3% vs. 5.7% (p=0.0001)
Any vascular event:	19.8% vs. 25.2% (p=0.0001)

The benefits of simvastatin were similar irrespective of age, gender, or baseline cholesterol. Benefit was even seen in those with an LDL-C of less than 3.0 mmol/L.

Adverse events
Simvastatin vs. Placebo:

Risk of myopathy:	0.01% per year
Muscle symptoms:	0.5% vs. 0.5% (p=NS)
Liver enzyme elevations (>4 ULN):	0.09% vs. 0.04% (p=NS)
Malignancy:	7.9% vs. 7.8% (p=NS)

Diabetic patients had a more pronounced benefit from simvastatin.
Vitamins did not significantly lower the rate of cardiovascular events.

Lipid Studies

Conclusion

Simvastatin 40 mg reduced mortality and major vascular events in high risk patients irrespective of their initial cholesterol levels.

Perspective

This was the first study to suggest that lowering LDL and total cholesterol levels with statin therapy should be a treatment goal for every patient at high risk for cardiovascular events irrespective of their baseline cholesterol levels. This concept ran contrary to the prevailing guidelines at the time. This trial showed that treating cholesterol to levels below current guideline recommendations for high risk patients could further benefit these patients irrespective of their baseline LDL-cholesterol levels. In fact, the real magnitude of benefit from statins may be even higher than reported considering that compliance was 85% in the statin arm, and 17% of placebo group were using non-study statins.

Along with HOPE (page 27), HPS was another definitive trial to refute the benefits of vitamins in vascular disease.

PROVE-IT-TIMI 22

Intensive versus Moderate Lipid Lowering with Statins after Acute Coronary Syndromes. Pravastatin or Atorvastatin Evaluation and Infection Therapy – Thrombolysis in Myocardial Infarction 22 Study.
New England Journal of Medicine 2004;350:1495-1504.

Study Question
Does aggressive lipid lowering to levels below that are recommended by the NCEP-ATP III Guidelines[13] further reduce major adverse cardiac events in patients presenting with ACS?

Methods
Double blind, randomized controlled trial which enrolled 4,162 patients presenting with an ACS.
Patients were randomized to pravastatin 40 mg or atorvastatin 80 mg daily.
Primary endpoint: a composite of death, MI, UA requiring re-hospitalization, revascularization (>30 days after randomization), and stroke.
Follow up was 18-36 months (mean of 24).

Results
At the end of the trial, median LDL levels in the atorvastatin arm were significantly lower than in the pravastatin group (1.6 mmol/L vs. 2.46 mmol/L p<0.001)

Atorvastatin vs. Pravastatin:
Primary endpoint:	22.4% vs. 26.3%	RRR 16%	(p=0.005)
Unstable Angina:	3.8% vs. 5.1%	RRR 29%	(p=0.02)
Revascularization:	16.3% vs. 18.8%	RRR 14%	(p=0.04)
Death or MI:	8.3% vs. 10%	RRR 18%	(p=0.06)
Death:	2.2% vs. 3.2%	RRR 28%	(p=0.07)
Stroke:	1.0% vs. 1.0%	NS	

The benefit of atorvastatin was consistent across all pre-specified subgroups and was seen as early as 30 days into the study.
Rates of drug discontinuation were not different between groups.

Adverse events
Atorvastatin vs. Pravastatin:
LE elevations (>3x ULN):	1.1% vs. 3.3%	(p<0.001)
Myalgia or CK elevation:	2.7% vs. 3.3%	(p=0.23)
Rhabdomyolysis:	none in either group.	

Lipid Studies

Conclusion

ACS patients treated with the high-dose atorvastatin received greater protection against death or major cardiovascular events than those treated with pravastatin 40 mg daily.

Perspective

This study (and the similarly designed but much smaller angiographic study, REVERSAL[14]) prompted a revision of the prevailing ACC/AHA Guidelines. The new version stated that in patients with an ACS it is reasonable to aggressively lower LDL levels to 1.8 mmol/L or less (i.e., the mean on-treatment LDL cholesterol level for the atorvastatin group).

The results of this study are remarkable in that the benefit of atorvastatin was seen despite the fact that the pravastatin group achieved the Guideline-recommended targets of LDL cholesterol (<2.5 mmol/L). In addition, the benefit of atorvastatin was demonstrated over and above the comprehensive secondary prevention and early invasive strategy that both groups received.

It is interesting to note that a subgroup analysis of this study showed that patients in the pravastatin group who achieved an LDL-cholesterol level of 1.6 mmol/L or less had the same benefits as the patients in the atorvastatin group. This suggests that the observed benefits are due to aggressive LDL-cholesterol lowering rather than being drug specific.

A similar trial, TNT[15] enrolled 10,001 patients with stable CHD and LDL-C levels of <3.4 mmol/L already tolerating 10 mg of atorvastatin. These patients were randomized to continue with 10 mg or to receive 80 mg of atorvastatin daily for 5 years. The latter group had a 22% RRR of CV death, nonfatal MI, resuscitation after cardiac arrest, or stroke (p<0.001). Overall mortality was not reduced.

One of the most frequent criticisms of recent statin-trials, like TNT and PROVE-IT, is that there is no statistically significant benefit in overall mortality. However, since previous studies such as the 4S (page 31), adequately powered to detect differences in mortality, have clearly demonstrated the mortality benefits associated with the use of statins randomizing patients with CVD to placebo is no longer ethical. Therefore, currently patients can only be involved in studies that treat both arms somewhat differently. In the 4S study that showed a mortality benefit, the LDL-C difference between the two arms was 38%, in PROVE-IT the difference was only about 30%, which still translated into a trend towards improved mortality. In TNT the LDL-difference of 22% in the two treatment arms resulted in a morbidity benefit only and in other studies like the ALLHAT-LLT[16], where the control arm was relatively aggressively treated the difference was only 9%, and therefore, no benefit was seen at all. If we still wanted to carry out trials that are powered to detect a mortality difference we would need mega trials with sample sizes in the range of 30,000-50,000, which is very challenging if at all possible. Thus, if we conduct trials in which the treatment arms are treated differently, but still in an ethically acceptable manner, comparative studies are likely only to demonstrate morbidity reductions. Furthermore, as evidenced by TNT and PEACE (page 29), current therapy results in such low mortality in both treatment and control groups that any further treatment benefit may be challenging to demonstrate.

13. NCEP *ATP III Guidelines: Circulation* 2002;106:3143-3421.
14. REVERSAL: *JAMA* 2004;291:1071-80.
15. TNT: *NEJM* 2005; 352:1425-1435.
16. ALLHAT-LLT: *JAMA* 2002; 288:2998-3007.

Hypertension

ALLHAT

Major Outcomes in High-Risk Hypertensive Patients Randomized to Angiotensin-converting Enzyme Inhibitor or Calcium Channel Blocker vs. Diuretic: The Antihypertensive and Lipid-Lowering Treatment to Prevent Heart Attack Trial.
JAMA 2002;288:2981-2997.

Study Question
What is the best pharmacologic regimen for the treatment of high blood pressure? What are the comparative benefits of different treatment regimens?

Methods
Double blind randomized controlled trial of 33,357 adults over the age of 55 years with HTN and one other CV risk factor.
Patients were randomized to one of three possible antihypertensives: ACE inhibitor (lisinopril) or CCB (amlodipine) or diuretic (chlorthalidone). Open label drugs (atenolol or reserpine or clonidine or hydralazine) could be added if patient were not at BP target (140/90 mmHg).
Mean follow up was 4.9 years.

Results
Blood pressure was significantly higher in the lisinopril (2 mmHg) and the amlodipine (0.8 mmHg) groups compared to chlorthalidone.

There was no difference between the 3 groups for the primary outcome (CV death or MI) or all cause mortality.

Primary outcome: CV death or nonfatal MI
Lisinopril vs. Chlorthalidone: 11.4% vs. 11.5% RR 0.99 (95% CI 0.91-1.08)
Amlodipine vs. Chlorthalidone: 11.3% vs. 11.5% RR 0.98 (95% CI 0.90-1.07)

Secondary outcomes:
Lisinopril vs. Chlorthalidone:
CV morbidity: 33.3% vs. 30.9%   RR 1.10 (95% CI 1.05-1.16)
Stroke: 6.3% vs. 5.6%   RR 1.15 (95% CI 1.02-1.30)
HF: 8.7% vs. 7.7%   RR 1.19 (95% CI 1.07-1.31)

Amlodipine vs. Chlorthalidone:
HF: 10.2% vs. 7.7%   RR 1.38 (95% CI 1.25-1.52)

Chlorthalidone vs. lisinopril:
New diabetes: 11.6% vs. 8.1%   ($p<0.001$)
New dyslipidemia: 14.4% vs. 12.8% ($p<0.001$)

Conclusion

The thiazide diuretic chlorthalidone is as good as other, more expensive, antihypertensives with respect to preventing cardiovascular outcomes. No excess in cardiovascular events was seen in the chlorthalidone group despite an excess of new diabetes and increase in lipid profiles.

Perspective

Initial antihypertensive studies showed important benefits of pharmacologic antihypertensive treatment compared to placebo. ALLHAT was the largest trial to address the question of which medications or combinations are better for the treatment of hypertension. The results of ALLHAT suggest that chlorthalidone strikes the best balance of efficacy and economy. Many experts believe that these results can be extrapolated to other thiazide diuretics such as hydrochlorothiazide. However, metabolic side effects, such as higher rates of new diabetes and new dyslipidemia, have tempered the enthusiasm to widely use them as first-line therapy. Nevertheless, thiazides remain very popular as second- or third-line agents in combination with other drugs, such as ACE inhibitors, ARBs and calcium channel blockers.

ALLHAT was criticized because it enrolled 35% African Americans, who respond to diuretics and CCBs better than to ACE inhibitors. Furthermore, drugs of the primary randomization could not be combined, and this restriction would not be consistent with current practice. Most patients with HTN are unable to achieve BP targets on one drug. Therefore, it is rather meaningless to compare individual medications to each other.

A few of the studies that addressed the same question are: LIFE, AASK, INVEST, INSIGHT, SCOPE, VALUE, and ASCOT[17-23]. None of these found any significant difference in hard outcomes between drug classes, but almost all showed minor differences that may become important for the individual patient.

The current evidence-based opinion is that some antihypertensive drugs may be better suited for certain individuals, but the most important goal remains to diagnose HTN and to significantly decrease BP in hypertensive patients.

17. LIFE: *Lancet* 2002;359:995-1003.
18. AASK: *JAMA* 2001;285:2719-28 and 2002;288:2421-31.
19. INVEST: *JAMA* 2003;290:2805-16.
20. INSIGHT: *Lancet* 2000;356:366-72.
21. SCOPE: *J Hypertension* 2003;21:875-86.
22. VALUE: *Lancet* 2004;363:2022-2031 and pages 2049-2051.
23. ASCOT: *Lancet* 2005;366:895-906.

Heart Failure/LV Dysfunction
SOLVD

Studies of Left Ventricular Dysfunction
New England Journal of Medicine 1991;325:293-302,
and *New England Journal of Medicine* 1992;327:685-691.

Study Question
Does enalapril reduce mortality and morbidity in patients with low ejection fraction with or without heart failure?

Methods
Double blind randomized controlled trial testing the effects of enalapril in the treatment and prevention of heart failure.
All 5,025 patients enrolled in the trial had LV systolic dysfunction (EF $\leq 35\%$). Patients were then stratified into two populations according to whether or not they had symptomatic heart failure. Patients with symptomatic heart failure formed the group which tested the enalapril treatment hypothesis and those without heart failure tested the enalapril prevention hypothesis.
Treatment arm: 2,569 patients, 90% NYHA II-III; follow up: 3.4 yrs.
Prevention arm: 4,228 patients; follow up of 37.4 months
All patients were randomized to enalapril 2.5-5 mg BID increased to 5-10 mg BID in 2 weeks or placebo.

Results
Treatment trial: Final mean dose of enalapril: 16.6 mg.

Enalapril vs. Placebo:
Mortality:	35.2% vs. 39.7%	RRR 16%	(p=0.0036)
Death or HF admission:	47.7% vs. 57.3%	RRR 26%	(p<0.0001)

Prevention trial:

Enalapril vs. Placebo:
Total mortality:	14.8% vs. 15.8%	RRR 8%	(p=0.3)
CV mortality:	12.6% vs. 14.1%	RRR 12%	(p=0.12)
Death and new HF:	29.8% vs. 38.6%	RRR 29%	(p<0.001)

Conclusion
Enalapril significantly reduced mortality in patients with chronic heart failure and LV dysfunction.

In patients with asymptomatic left ventricular dysfunction there was only a trend towards reduced CV mortality but the combined endpoint of death and hospitalization for HF was significantly reduced by enalapril.

Perspective

A series of similar studies conducted with different ACE inhibitors (SAVE, AIRE, TRACE, V-HeFT II, CONSENSUS[24-28] etc.) showed very similar results. ACE inhibitors significantly decreased mortality and heart failure admissions in patients with chronic heart failure as well as in post-MI LVD with or without HF. Therefore, ACE inhibitors became first-line therapy and remain the mainstay of treatment in systolic heart failure and in asymptomatic LV dysfunction both post MI as well as in non-ischemic cardiomyopathy, although there is limited data in this group.

24. SAVE: *NEJM* 1992;327:669-677.
25. AIRE: *Lancet* 1993;342:821-8.
26. TRACE : *NEJM* 1995;333:1670-6.
27. V-HeFT II: *NEJM* 1991;325:303-10.
28. CONSENSUS: *NEJM* 1987;316:1429-35.

DIG

The Effect of Digoxin on Mortality and Morbidity in Patients with Heart Failure. The Digitalis Investigation Group.
New England Journal of Medicine 1997;336:525-533.

Study Question
Does digoxin improve mortality and morbidity in heart failure?

Methods
Double blind RCT in which patients with HF and LVEF ≤45% were randomized to digoxin (median dose, 0.25 mg daily) or placebo in addition to diuretics and ACE inhibitors (average follow up, 37 months). In a secondary trial of patients with heart failure and EF>45%, 988 patients were randomly assigned to digoxin or placebo. Only patients in normal sinus rhythm were randomized.

Results
Digoxin vs. Placebo:
Overall mortality:	34.8% vs. 35.1%	(p=0.80)
Death due to worsening HF:	11.6% vs. 13.2%	(RRR 12%, p= 0.06)
Hospitalization for worsening HF:	26.8% vs. 34.7 %	(RRR 28%, p<0.001)

Subgroup analysis demonstrated that patients with worse heart failure received the most benefit from digoxin.

Adverse events
Digoxin vs. Placebo:
VT or cardiac arrest: 4.2% vs. 4.3%   (p=NS)

Conclusion
Digoxin did not reduce overall mortality, but it reduced the rate of hospitalization for worsening HF.

Perspective
Over the past 15 years there has been substantial enthusiasm for the use of intravenous and oral positive inotropes to improve symptoms and outcomes in patients with systolic heart failure. To date almost all studies of potent inotropes have demonstrated improved symptoms at the cost of increased complications, including mortality.

While the DIG study failed to demonstrate a mortality benefit it did achieve important quality of life endpoints such as improved HF symptoms and reduced hospital admissions. In the current era of evidence based practice, any medical therapy must show a reduction in 'hard' cardiovascular endpoints to gain widespread endorsement. That being said, digoxin remains useful in patients with ongoing symptoms of congestion.

CHARM

Candesartan in Heart Failure Assessment of Reduction in Mortality and Morbidity
CHARM-Overall: *Lancet* 2003; 362: 759-766.
CHARM-Added: *Lancet* 2003; 362: 767-771.
CHARM-Alternative: *Lancet* 2003; 362: 772-776
CHARM-Preserved: *Lancet* 2003; 362: 777-781.

Study Question

1) Does the angiotensin II receptor antagonist candesartan improve heart failure and mortality in patients with heart failure who are already on ACE inhibitors?
2) Can ACE-intolerant heart failure patients tolerate candesartan and does it improve on their cardiovascular outcomes?
3) Does candesartan improve cardiovascular outcomes of patients with heart failure and preserved LV systolic function?

Methods

CHARM-Overall was a double blind randomized controlled trial of 7,601 patients with chronic heart failure. All enrolled patients were randomized to candesartan or placebo. Three component studies were carried out simultaneously that stratified patients according to:

1. Concomitant use of ACE inhibitor   (**CHARM-Added**, n = 2,548)
2. Intolerance to ACE inhibitor   (**CHARM-Alternative**, n = 2,028)
3. Preserved ejection fraction   (**CHARM-Preserved**, n = 3,023)

Follow up was at least 2 years.
The primary endpoint of the main trial was all-cause mortality.
The primary endpoint for each sub-study was CV death or hospital admission for CHF.

Results

CHARM – Overall
Candesartan vs. Placebo:
Death: 23% vs. 25%   RR 0.91 (95% CI 0.83-1.00, p=0.055)
CV death: 18% vs. 20%   RR 0.88 (95% CI 0.79-0.97, p=0.012)
Admissions for CHF: 20% vs. 24%   (p<0.0001)

More patients discontinued candesartan than placebo because of renal dysfunction, hypotension and hyperkalaemia.

CHARM-Added
Candesartan vs. Placebo:
CV death/HF hospitalization: 37.9% vs. 42.3% RR 0.85 (95% CI 0.75-0.96, p=0.011)
CV death: 23.7% vs. 27.3% RR 0.84 (95% CI 0.72-0.98, p=0.029)
Admissions for CHF: 24.2% vs. 28.0% RR 0.83 (95% CI 0.71-0.96, p=0.01)

Similar results in all predefined subgroups, including patients also receiving baseline beta blocker treatment.

CHARM-Alternative
Candesartan vs. Placebo:
CV death/HF hospitalization: 33% vs. 40% RR 0.77 (95% CI 0.67-0.89, p=0.0004)
CV death: 21.6% vs. 24.8% RR 0.85 (95% CI 0.71-1.02, p=0.072)
HF hospitalization: 20.4% vs. 28.2% RR 0.68 (95% CI 0.57-0.81, p<0.0001)

Study-drug discontinuation rates were similar to placebo.

CHARM-Preserved
Candesartan vs. Placebo:
CV death/HF hospitalization: 22% vs. 24.3% RR 0.89 (95% CI 0.77-1.03, p=0.118)
CV death: 11.2% vs. 11.3% RR 0.99 (95% CI 0.80-1.22, p=NS)
Admissions for CHF: 15.9% vs. 18.3% RR 0.85 (95% CI 0.72-1.01, p=0.072)

Conclusion
Candesartan significantly reduced the combined endpoint of CV death and hospital admissions for HF in the overall CHARM population, and it was especially effective in patients with decreased EF. The addition of candesartan to an ACE inhibitor led to a reduction in the combined endpoint in patients with CHF and reduced LVEF. Candesartan prevented HF admissions in patients with HF irrespective of LVEF. The drug was generally well tolerated.

Perspective
CHARM was the largest study to date to assess the efficacy and safety of an angiotensin-receptor blocker (ARB) in HF. However, the results of the CHARM-Overall program are difficult to interpret as CHARM-Overall consists of three trials with three distinct HF patient populations. CHARM-Added demonstrated

Heart Failure/LV Dysfunction

a reduction of the combined endpoint of mortality and HF admission with candesartan. However, clinical application of this combination has been hampered by the lack of consistently positive results of other ARB-studies, like Val-HeFT[29] and VALIANT[30], which did not show similarly impressive improvement with the combination of ACE inhibitors and another ARB, valsartan. CHARM provoked a debate as to what extent the treatment effects of ARBs exhibit a class effect. A sensible approach is to use the specific drugs in doses that have been shown to reduce hard clinical endpoints in large trials. Therefore, results of CHARM-Added can be applied to clinical practice as long as there is appropriate monitoring for side-effects such as hyperkalemia.

The issue of hyperkalemia should not be underestimated in light of the impressive results of the RALES study (see page 46) which demonstrated mortality benefit of spironolactone in addition to ACE inhibition in heart failure patients. The benefit of spironolactone was achieved at the expense of slight increases in potassium levels. Given that many heart failure patients will already be on spironolactone and ACE inhibitor, the addition of ARB requires vigilant electrolyte monitoring.

Based on a retrospective analysis, the Val-HeFT Study[26] suggested that the triple combination of an ACE inhibitor, an ARB and a beta blocker might have detrimental effects. CHARM-Added refuted this concern.

CHARM-Alternative confirmed that candesartan is both safe and effective in ACE-intolerant patients even if they had ACE-induced angioedema.

Although the CHARM-Preserved arm did not yield a significant mortality benefit it is still the first trial to show that an ARB is effective in patients with heart failure and normal left ventricular function.

29. Val-HeFT: *NEJM* 2001;345:1667-75.
30. VALIANT: *NEJM* 2003; 349:1893-1906.

Heart Failure/LV Dysfunction

RALES

Randomized Aldactone Evaluation Study.
New England Journal of Medicine 1999;341:709-717.

Study Question
Does aldactone reduce mortality in patients with advanced heart failure who are already on standard medical therapy including ACE inhibitors?

Methods
Double blind randomized controlled trial of 1,663 patients with NYHA II-IV HF and LVEF $\leq 35\%$.
Patients randomized to spironolactone 25 mg daily or placebo.
Primary endpoint: death from all causes.

Results
The trial was discontinued early, at 24 months, due to a clear benefit of spironolactone.

Aldactone vs. Placebo:
All cause mortality: 34.5% vs. 45.9% RR 0.70 (95% CI 0.60-0.82, p<0.001)
Death due to HF: 15.5% vs. 22.5% RR 0.64 (95% CI 0.51-0.80, p<0.001)
Sudden death: 10.0 % vs. 13.1% RR 0.71 (95% CI 0.54-0.95, p=0.02)
HF hospitalizations: 215 episodes vs. 300 episodes RR 0.65 (95% CI 0.54-0.77, p<0.001)

Adverse events
Aldactone vs. Placebo:
Gynecomastia or breast pain in men: 10% vs. 1% (p<0.001)
Hyperkalemia was rare in both groups.

Conclusion
The aldosterone receptor-blocker spironolactone, in addition to standard therapy, substantially reduced the risk of morbidity and mortality among patients with severe systolic HF.

Perspective
Rarely in the scientific community has a single study affected practice and guidelines without confirmatory work and replication of the results. With the RALES study, spironolactone therapy became widely accepted and implemented with little hesitation because the trial showed an impressive mortality reduction as well as significant improvement in all the other cardiac endpoints. In addition, spironolactone is inexpensive and does not have a significant hypotensive effect.

The background heart failure therapy among RALES patients was up to the then current standards with over 90% of patients receiving an ACE inhibitor, 100% a loop diuretic and 75% digoxin. Only 10% of the patients were on a beta blocker. However, beta blockers exert their beneficial effects via a different mechanism.

The most significant concerns that have arisen from the "real world application" of spironolactone in the treatment of severe heart failure stem from the significantly increased incidence of hyperkalemia and worsening renal function.

MERIT-HF

Effect of Metoprolol CR/XL in Chronic Heart Failure: Metoprolol CR/XL Randomized Intervention Trial in Congestive Heart Failure.
Lancet 1999;353:2001-2007.

Study Question
Does metoprolol therapy reduce mortality in patients with systolic heart failure due to ischemic cardiomyopathy?

Methods
Double blind RCT of 3,991 adults, aged 40-80 years with HF (LVEF <40%) secondary to IHD. Non-ischemic cardiomyopathy was excluded.
Patients were randomized to metoprolol CR/XL (target dose 200 mg/day) vs. placebo. Administration of metoprolol started at 12.5 mg or 25 mg/d and doubled every 2 weeks until the target or the maximum tolerated dose was achieved.

Results
The study was stopped early because of significant mortality benefit with metoprolol. Mean follow up was one year.
Mean daily dose of the study drug was 159 mg at the end of the trial.
90% of patients were also on ACE inhibitors and diuretics.

Metoprolol vs. Placebo:
All cause annual mortality: 7.2% vs. 11% RR 0.66 (95% CI 0.53–0.81, $p=0.00009$)
CV death: RR 0.62 (95% CI 0.50–0.78, $p=0.00003$)
Sudden cardiac death: 4% vs. 6.7%   RR 0.59 (95% CI 0.45–0.78, $p=0.0002$)
Death from HF: 1.5% vs. 2.9% RR 0.51 (95% CI 0.33–0.79, $p=0.0023$).

Conclusion
There is a highly significant mortality benefit with metoprolol treatment in patients with heart failure secondary to ischemic cardiomyopathy.

Perspective
For many years the use of negative chronotropic and inotropic agents such as a beta blocker in heart failure was considered to be absolutely contraindicated. Further understanding of the pathophysiological mechanism of the negative feedback spiral with the body's own compensation leading to progressive congestion and worsening heart failure allowed expansion of therapeutic

options to include agents such as beta blockers.

MERIT-HF was the first moderate sized trial to demonstrate a mortality advantage of beta blockers in ischemic heart failure in patients with an EF <40%. This work was followed up by a host of trials (CIBIS II, COPERNICUS, COMET[31-33] etc.) in both ischemic and non-ischemic HF patient populations that have solidified the use of beta blockers in all patients with systolic heart failure. It is important to recognize that beta blocker therapy should be initiated once patients have achieved clinical stability with other appropriate heart failure medications and the dose should be carefully titrated.

31. CIBIS II: *Lancet* 1999;353:9-13.
32. COPERNICUS: *NEJM* 2001;344:1651-8.
33. COMET: *Lancet* 2003;362:7-13.

Heart Failure/LV Dysfunction/Arrhythmias
MADIT-II

Prophylactic Implantation of a Defibrillator in Patients with Myocardial Infarction and Reduced Ejection Fraction. The Multicenter Automatic Defibrillator Implantation Trial II Investigators.
New England Journal of Medicine 2002;346:877-883.

Study Question
Does ICD implantation improve mortality in patients who have severe LV dysfunction following an AMI but no history of ventricular arrhythmias?

Methods
Randomized controlled trial designed to evaluate the effect of an implantable defibrillator on survival in 1,232 adults with IHD and EF<30%.
(Excluded: NYHA IV, active CHF, MI within 1 month, or revascularization within 3 months).
Open label 3:2 randomization to Automated Implantable Cardiac Defibrillator (AICD) implantation versus medical therapy.
Average follow up 20 months.

Results
Patients in both groups were generally on good therapy for IHD and HF (67% on ACE-I, 70% on beta blocker, 67% on statins).
Average LV ejection fraction: 23%.

AICD vs. Medical Therapy
Overall mortality: 14.2% vs. 19.8% RR 0.69 (95% CI 0.51-0.93, p=0.016)
The mortality benefit was only seen after 9 months of AICD implantation.

Subgroup analysis
  Benefit only if QRS >150msec.

Adverse events of AICD
  Lead problems 1.8%.
  Infections: 0.7%.
  Development of HF (AICD vs. medical therapy): 19.9% vs. 14.9% (p=0.09).

Conclusion
AICD implantation confers significant mortality benefit in patients with a prior MI and advanced LV dysfunction.

Perspective

This was the first large trial to show mortality benefit of ICD therapy in patients identified purely by LVEF, QRS width, and functional class. The mortality benefit was similar no matter how long after the index myocardial infarction the ICD was implanted.

There was a non-significant trend to greater heart failure admissions in the AICD group compared to the medical therapy group. The authors propose that by preventing sudden cardiac death, patients survive longer and consequently develop more complications related to their heart failure. In addition, the effects of repeated shocks and chronic ventricular pacing on heart function are not well understood.

Cost-effectiveness remains a problem due to the high cost and limited lifespan of the AICD device. In more recent studies, such as the SCD-HeFT[34], a less expensive, single lead "shock only" ICD was used and that may turn out to be more cost effective.

34. SCD-HeFT: *NEJM* 2005;352:225-37.

Arrhythmias Including Atrial Fibrillation

CAST

Cardiac Arrhythmia Suppression Trial.
New England Journal of Medicine 1989;321:406-412.

Study Question
Does suppressing ventricular ectopy with class I antiarrhythmic medications improve mortality in patients post myocardial infarction?

Method
Double blind randomized controlled trial of 2,309 patients with asymptomatic or mildly symptomatic ventricular arrhythmia after myocardial infarction. Patients were randomized to receive one of three Class I antiarrhythmic agents: encainide, flecainide, or moricizine or placebo.
75% had initial suppression of ventricular ectopy demonstrated by Holter monitor and then were randomized to receive active drug or placebo. Average follow up was 10 months.

Results
This trial was stopped early due to an excess mortality in the treatment arms.
Encanide or Flecanide vs. Placebo:
Death from arrhythmia: 4.5% vs. 1.2%   RR 3.6   (95% CI 1.7-8.5)
Total mortality: 7.7% vs. 3.0%   RR 2.5   (95% CI 1.6-4.5)

Conclusion
Encainide and flecainide both increased mortality and therefore should not be used in the treatment of patients with asymptomatic or minimally symptomatic ventricular arrhythmia after MI, even though these drugs may be effective initially in suppressing ventricular arrhythmia.

Perspective
Scientific rigour requires careful interrogation of associations of clinical phenomena in contrast to cause and effect relationships. It had been well established that following acute myocardial infarction, complex ventricular arrhythmias were associated with worse outcomes, including arrhythmic death. Anti-arrhythmic agents were shown to suppress these dysrhythmias and therefore it was believed that these agents would prevent arrhythmic death. The CAST trial provided a very important warning that anti-arrhythmic drugs may increase mortality and therefore their safety must be tested in other patient populations as well. This trial was the first of a series of studies that led physicians to use anti-arrhythmic medications less frequently, especially in acute myocardial infarction, but also across a broad spectrum of cardiovascular disease.

AFASAK

Placebo Controlled, Randomised Trial of Warfarin and Aspirin for Prevention of Thromboembolic Complications in Chronic Atrial Fibrillation.
Lancet 1989;333:175-179.

Study Question
What is the best treatment strategy to prevent thromboembolic complications of atrial fibrillation?

Methods
Randomized controlled trial of 1,007 adults with non-rheumatic atrial fibrillation.
Patients were randomized to one of three groups 1) open label warfarin (target INR 2.8-4.2), 2) aspirin 75 mg, or 3) placebo.

Results
Significant age differences between groups: warfarin (72.8yrs), placebo (74.6yrs), and ASA (75.1yrs).
Warfarin-treated patients were within INR target 42% of the time and an INR of 2.4-4.2 73% of the time.
Only 1 out of 4 ischemic infarcts occurred with a therapeutic INR.
38% of patients in the warfarin arm stopped medication due to bleeding complications or frustration with frequent bloodwork.

Primary endpoint: thromboembolic complication (stroke or TIA or arterial thromboembolism):

Warfarin vs. ASA vs. Placebo:
Stroke or TIA or arterial thromboembolism: 1.5% vs. 6.0% vs. 6.3% ($p<0.05$)
Vascular death: 0.9% vs. 3.6% vs. 4.5 % ($p<0.02$)
Annual thromboembolic event rate: 2.0% vs. 5.5% vs. 5.5% (p not given)

Adverse Effects
Warfarin vs. ASA vs. Placebo:
Bleeding events: 6.2% vs. 0.6% vs. 0% ($p=0.001$)

Conclusion
Anticoagulation with warfarin (INR 2.8-4.2) is significantly more effective than aspirin or placebo in preventing thromboembolic complications of atrial fibrillation.

Perspective

This was the first trial to test the theory that anticoagulation or antiplatelet therapy could reduce the risk of thromboembolic complications in atrial fibrillation. Although the results seemed to unequivocally prove the role of warfarin in this setting, unblinded interpretation of thromboembolic events in the warfarin group could have led to the underestimation of the number of events in the warfarin group.

However, numerous follow up studies[35-39] established that warfarin cannot be replaced by aspirin in the thromboembolic prevention in atrial fibrillation. As well, these studies confirmed that an INR 2-3 is as effective as a higher INR in preventing thromboembolic complications without increasing the bleeding risk as much as a higher INR.

These studies also identified the risk factors that are associated with a higher risk of thromboembolism in AF, such as prior stroke or TIA, LVD or HF, HTN, valvular disease, age >75 years. Other characteristics associated with thromboembolism such as age 65-75 years, DM, thyrotoxicosis and CAD were found to be risk factors in some but not in all studies.

35. SPAF I: *Circulation* 1991;84:527-39
36. SPAF II: *Lancet* 1994;343:687-91.
37. BAATAF: *NEJM* 1990;323:1505-11.
38. CAFA: *J Am Coll Cardiol* 1991;18:349-55.
39. SPINAF: *NEJM* 1992;327:1406-12.

AFFIRM

A Comparison of Rate Control and Rhythm Control in Patients with Atrial Fibrillation. Atrial Fibrillation Follow up Investigation of Rhythm Management Investigators.
New England Journal of Medicine 2002;347:1825-33.

Study Question
What is the preferred management strategy for patients with atrial fibrillation: rate control or rhythm control?

Methods
Randomized controlled trial of 4,060 adults over the age of 65 with recurrent atrial fibrillation.
Patients were randomized to rate or rhythm control. Appropriate rate control was defined as HR<80 bpm at rest, and <110 bpm on a 6-minute walk test. Physicians could use their discretion as to the selection of medical regimen. Rhythm control approach included cardioversion if necessary and an anti-arrhythmic of the attending physician's choice. Anticoagulation could be stopped, if patients appeared to be in sinus rhythm for 4-12 weeks.
Mean follow up was 3.5 years.

Results
Most commonly used anti-arrhythmic medications included amiodarone, sotalol, and propafenone, and 62.5% of patients achieved rhythm control at 5 year follow up.

Most commonly used rate control medications include digoxin, beta blocker, and CCB, and 80% of patients achieved rate control.

Rate vs. Rhythm:
All cause mortality:	25.9% vs. 26.7%	(p=0.08)
Ischemic stroke*:	5.5% vs. 7.1%	(p=0.79)
Warfarin use:	90% vs. 70%	
Hospitalization:	73% vs. 80.1%	(p<0.001)

Adverse events
Rate vs. Rhythm:
Torsades de pointes:	0.2% vs. 0.8%	(p=0.007)
Sustained VT:	0.7% vs. 0.6%	(p=0.44)

*Two thirds of ischemic strokes in both groups occurred when warfarin was being held or when the patient's INR was sub-therapeutic.

Conclusion

Management of atrial fibrillation with the rhythm-control strategy offers no survival advantage over the rate-control strategy. Moreover, there are potential advantages, such as a lower risk of adverse drug effects, with the rate-control strategy. Anticoagulation should be continued in this group of high-risk patients regardless of the selected treatment strategy.

Perspective

The AFFIRM trial results reassured clinicians that aggressive rate-control was a reasonable alternative to rhythm control. Also, antiarrhythmic drugs that were given more often in the rhythm control group have been shown to adversely affect survival especially in patients with IHD, whereas beta blockers, given more often in the rate-control group do not have such an adverse effect and may be even beneficial.

The majority of strokes in both groups occurred when anticoagulation was held or was sub-therapeutic, which underscores the dangers of stopping anticoagulation in patients with paroxysmal atrial fibrillation even if they appear to maintain normal sinus rhythm.

Despite these considerations practitioners are frequently reminded that a minority of patients cannot tolerate atrial fibrillation well and for these patients rhythm control (with anticoagulation) remains the best option.

Hormone Replacement Therapy
WOMEN'S HEALTH INITIATIVE (WHI)

Risks and Benefits of Estrogen Plus Progestin in Healthy Postmenopausal Women. Principal Results from the Women's Health Initiative Randomized Controlled Trial.
JAMA 2002;288:321-333.

Study Question
Is hormone replacement therapy a safe way to reduce cardiovascular events in postmenopausal women?

Methods
Double blind randomized controlled trial of 16,608 postmenopausal women (50-79 years old) with an intact uterus.
Patients were randomized to hormone replacement (0.625 mg estrogen + 2.5 mg medroxyprogesterone) or placebo.
Follow up 5.2 years (8.5 planned).
Primary endpoint: nonfatal MI and CHD death.
Primary adverse outcome: invasive breast cancer.

Results
The trial was stopped early due to excess risk of invasive breast cancer in the HRT group.
Hazard ratio of main outcomes:

HRT vs. Placebo:

Total Mortality:	0.98 (95% CI 0.82-1.18)
Coronary heart disease:	1.29 (95% CI 1.02-1.63)
Breast cancer:	1.26 (95% CI 1.00-1.59)
Stroke:	1.41 (95% CI 1.07-1.85)
Pulmonary Embolism:	2.13 (95% CI 1.39-3.25)
Colorectal Cancer:	0.63 (95% CI 0.43-0.92)
Endometrial Cancer:	0.83 (95% CI 0.47-1.47)
Hip Fracture:	0.66 (95% CI 0.45-0.98)

The net effect of estrogen and progestin therapy (per 10,000 person-years) was 5 fewer colorectal cancers and 5 fewer hip fractures at the expense of 7 excess CHD events, 8 excess strokes, 8 excess pulmonary emboli and 8 more invasive breast carcinomas.

The adverse cardiovascular outcomes of HRT became evident soon after randomization whereas the excess risk for breast cancer emerged after about 4 years.

The increased risks associated with HRT were present across all racial/ethnic and age strata.

When the analysis was repeated looking only at patients actually taking HRT (i.e., on-treatment analysis) it showed even higher risks for adverse outcomes than the original intention to treat analysis.

Conclusion

HRT treatment in postmenopausal women is associated with significant adverse cardiovascular, thromboembolic and malignant events. These data do not support the use of HRT for the prevention of cardiovascular outcomes.

Perspective

This study put an end to another age-old debate about the usefulness of HRT in preventing cardiovascular events. While there were significant benefits seen regarding hip fractures, almost all the other main outcomes showed increased risks with hormone replacement. In addition, during the time this study was being conducted, new therapies for osteoporosis were identified (i.e., bisphosphonates) that were both safe and effective, rendering HRT obsolete for the indication of osteoporosis prevention. This trial could not distinguish between the effects of estrogen and progestin. The adverse effects of progestin were initially thought to be more important for breast cancer and atherosclerotic diseases than estrogen. However, the final results of the WHI estrogen-only trial confirmed that in 10,739 women who had had a previous hysterectomy, the benefits of estrogen therapy (specifically a reduction in bone fracture) was offset by an increase in stroke and venous thromboembolic events. However, unlike in the main trial, in this patient population there was no increased risk for breast cancer found.[40]

40. WHI Estrogen only Study: *Arch Intern Med* 2006;166:357-65.

Diabetes and the Heart

UKPDS-38

Tight Blood Pressure Control and Risk of Macrovascular and Microvascular Complications in Type 2 Diabetes.
British Medical Journal 1998;317:703-713.

Study Question
Does tight blood pressure control reduce vascular complications of diabetes mellitus?

Methods
Double blind randomized controlled trial of 1,148 patients with type II DM and HTN (>150/85 mmHg)
Exclusion: independent indication for strict BP control (prior stroke, accelerated HTN, CHF, renal failure) or independent indication for a beta blocker (current angina or MI within 1 year).
Patients were randomized to tight BP control (<150/85) using captopril or atenolol vs. less tight control (180/105 mmHg) with avoidance of ACE inhibitors or beta blockers.
Median follow up was 8.4 years.

Results

Tight BP Control vs. Less Tight BP Control:
BP reduction:	144/82 vs. 154/87 mmHg	(p<0.0001)
Stroke:	11% vs. 65%	(p=0.013)
Diabetes mortality*:	6% vs. 51%	(p=0.019)
Visual deterioration:	7% vs. 70%	(p=0.004)
Microvascular endpoints[†]:	11% vs. 56%	(p=0.0092)

*Diabetes mortality included death due to: MI, sudden cardiac death, stroke, PVD, renal disease, hyper/hypoglycemia)
[†]Microvascular endpoints included: retinopathy requiring photocoagulation, vitreous hemorrhage, and renal failure)

Conclusion
Blood pressure control to a level of <150/80 amongst diabetics has wide ranging benefits in stroke and microvascular outcomes.

FURTHER UKPDS STUDIES

UKPDS 39

BMJ 1998:317;713-720 – BP lowering with captopril or atenolol was similarly effective in reducing the incidence of diabetic complications suggesting that BP reduction in itself may be more important than the treatment used.

UKPDS 33

Lancet 1998;352:837-853 – Intensive blood-glucose control by either sulphonylureas or insulin substantially decreased the risk of microvascular complications. Results regarding macrovascular disease were less impressive although the risk of MI was almost significantly reduced (p=0.052).

UKPDS 34

Lancet 1998;352:854-865 – Intensive glucose control with metformin appeared to decrease the risk of diabetes related endpoints (death, stroke, etc.) in overweight diabetic patients. It was also associated with less weight gain and fewer hypoglycaemic attacks than insulin and sulphonylureas, therefore this was the study that established metformin as first-line pharmacological therapy in these patients.

Perspective

The UKPDS studies provided the first evidence that tight BP and glucose control may not only be logical and prudent, but that they also decrease the risk of diabetic complications. The magnitude of benefit, however, was not all that impressive likely due to the fact that each individual UKPDS study attempted to control only one risk factor (i.e., diabetes **or** hypertension) and lipid control was not systematically addressed at all. Current Diabetes Guidelines have used the UKPDS trials, among others, as a basis for the prevention of vascular complications using tight blood pressure control as well as tight glucose and lipid control.

Additional References

1. ISIS-2: *Lancet* 1986;328:57-66.
2. COMMIT-CCS 2 – clopidogrel randomization: *Lancet* 2005;366:1607-21.
3. FRISC II: *Lancet* 1999;354:708-15.
4. ESSENCE: *NEJM* 1997;337:447-52.
5. TIMI 11B: *Circulation* 1999;100:1593-1601.
6. ICTUS: *NEJM* 2005;353:1095-1104.
7. ISAR-COOL: *JAMA* 2003;290:1593-9.
8. ISAR-REACT 2: *JAMA* 2006;295:1531:8.
9. INTERHEART: *Lancet* 2004;364:937-952.
10. IMAGINE: presented at the European Society of Cardiology Congress, Stockholm, Sweden, August, 2005.
11. EUROPA: *Lancet* 2003;362:782-788.
12. Yusuf: *N Engl J Med.* 2005;352:937-8.
13. NCEP ATP III Lipid Guidelines: *Circulation* 2002;106:3143-3421.
14. REVERSAL: *JAMA* 2004;291:1071-80.
15. TNT: *NEJM* 2005;352:1425-1435.
16. ALLHAT-LLT: *JAMA* 2002;288:2998-3007.
17. LIFE: *Lancet* 2002;359:995-1003.
18. AASK: *JAMA* 2001;285:2719-28 and 2002;288:2421-31.
19. INVEST: *JAMA* 2003;290:2805-16.
20. INSIGHT: *Lancet* 2000;356:366-72.
21. SCOPE: *J Hypertension* 2003;21:875-86.
22. VALUE: *Lancet* 2004;363:2022-2031 and pages 2049-2051.
23. ASCOT: *Lancet* 2005;366:895-906.
24. SAVE: *NEJM* 1992;327:669-677.
25. AIRE: *Lancet* 1993;342:821-8.
26. TRACE: *NEJM* 1995;333:1670-6.
27. V-HeFT II: *NEJM* 1991;325:303-10.
28. CONSENSUS: *NEJM* 1987;316:1429-35.
29. Val-HeFT: *NEJM* 2001;345:1667-75.
30. VALIANT: *NEJM* 2003;349:1893-1906.
31. CIBIS II: *Lancet* 1999;353:9-13.
32. COPERNICUS: *NEJM* 2001;344:1651-8.
33. COMET : *Lancet* 2003;362:7-13.
34. SCD-HeFT: *NEJM* 2005;352:225-37.
35. SPAF I: *Circulation* 1991;84:527-39.
36. SPAF II: *Lancet* 1994;343:687-91.
37. BAATAF: *NEJM* 1990;323:1505-11.
38. CAFA: *J Am College Cardiol* 1991;18:349-55.
39. SPINAF: *NEJM* 1992;327:1406-12.
40. WHI Estrogen only Study: *Arch Intern Med* 2006;166:357-65.

Notes

Notes